Organic Body Scrubs

30 Organic Body Scrubs for Beautiful and Glowing Skin

Disclaimer and Terms of Use:

Effort has been made to ensure that the information in this book is accurate and complete, however, the author and the publisher do not warrant the accuracy of the information, text and graphics contained within the book due to the rapidly changing nature of science, research, known and unknown facts and internet. The Author and the publisher do not hold any responsibility for errors, omissions or contrary interpretation of the subject matter herein. This book is presented solely for motivational and informational purposes only.

Table of Contents

Introduction

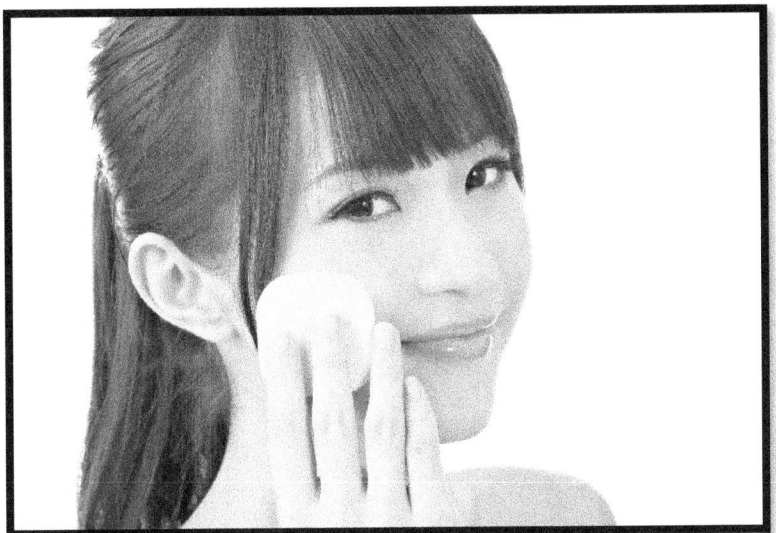

If you've ever been to a beauty boutique store or have paid a small fortune for organic beauty products at a spa, you will be glad to know that you never have to do it again. Making your own organic scrubs at home is easier than you might think – you just need a few simple ingredients. Homemade body scrubs can help to exfoliate and moisturize your skin, helping to relieve itchiness and redness from various skin conditions like eczema and psoriasis – even sunburn. And don't forget about the delicate skin on your lips – homemade lip scrubs can help to moisturize chapped lips and leave them smooth and softer than ever. If you are ready to try making your own organic body scrubs at home, this book is the perfect place to start!

Organic Body Scrub Recipes

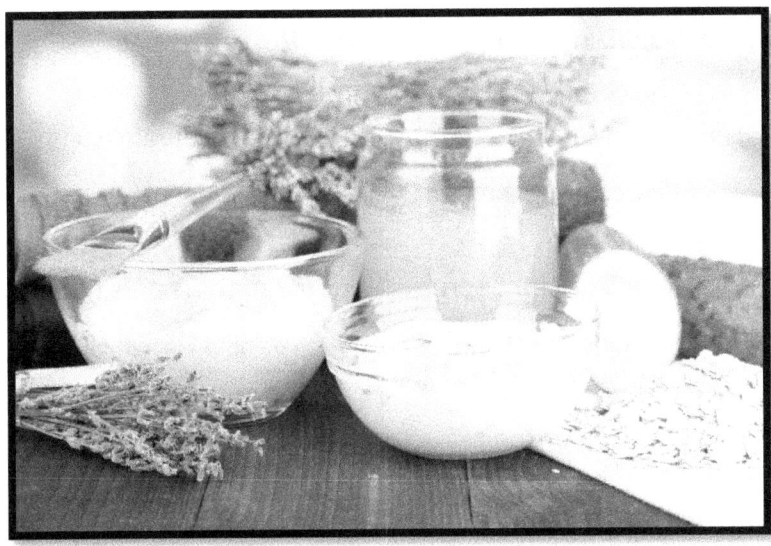

<u>Recipes Included in this Book</u>:

Easy Brown Sugar Scrub

Soothing Vanilla
Lavender Scrub

Cinnamon Honey Lip
Scrub

Energizing Coffee Scrub

Pumpkin Honey Scrub

Lemon Coconut Lip
Scrub

Avocado Grapefruit
Scrub

Refreshing Lemon Scrub

Mint Chocolate Java Lip
Scrub

Chocolate Cake Scrub

Green Tea and Citrus
Scrub

Spiced Chai Scrub

Peppermint Lip Scrub

Coffee Coconut Sugar Scrub

Coconut Vanilla Sugar Scrub

Mint and Pepper Scrub

Honey Lime Lip Scrub

Moisturizing Banana Scrub

Rosemary Lemon Salt Scrub

Tropical Mango Scrub

Ripe Tomato Sugar Scrub

Skin-Soothing Oatmeal Scrub

Minty Sugar Lip Scrub

Mint and Grapefruit Scrub

Orange Sea Salt Scrub

Exfoliating Berry Lip Scrub

Vanilla Brown Sugar Scrub

Brown Sugar Banana Scrub

Lemon Raspberry Sugar Scrub

Lavender Sea Salt Scrub

Easy Brown Sugar Scrub

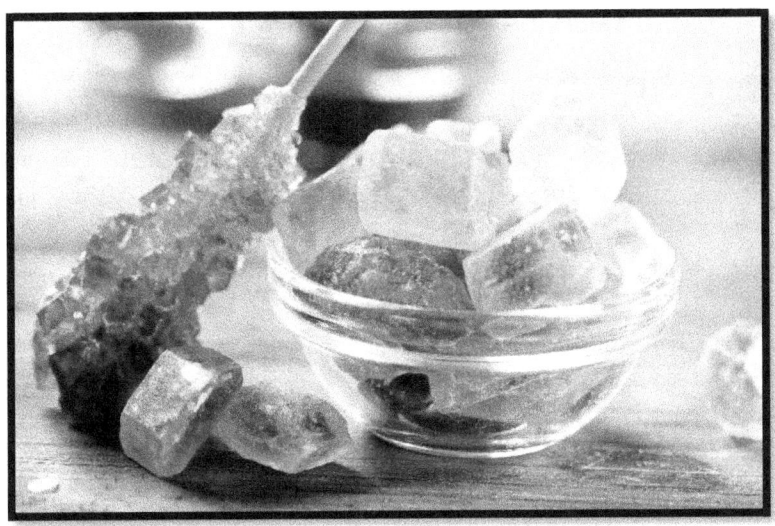

Ingredients:

½ cup organic brown sugar

¼ cup organic coconut oil

10 to 15 drops essential oils (optional)

Instructions:

1. Combine the sugar and coconut oil in a glass jar.
2. Stir the ingredients until well combined.
3. Add a few drops of your favorite essential oil to scent the scrub – stir well.
4. Place the lid tightly on the jar and store at room temperature until ready to use.

5. To use the scrub, dampen your skin in the shower then scrub with 1 tablespoon of the scrub mixture.

6. Rinse the scrub away with warm water to leave your skin feeling refreshed.

Soothing Vanilla Lavender Scrub

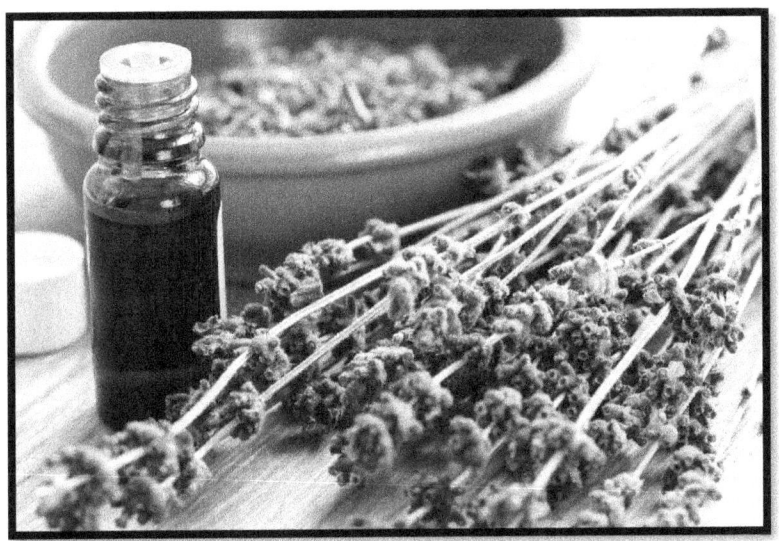

Ingredients:

2 cups organic raw sugar

1 cup organic avocado oil

1 teaspoon organic vanilla extract

1 tablespoon organic dried lavender

10 to 12 drops organic lavender essential oil

Instructions:

1. Combine the sugar and oil in a medium mixing bowl.
2. Stir the ingredients until well combined.
3. Add the remaining ingredients and stir well then transfer to a glass jar.
4. Place the lid tightly on the jar and store at room temperature until ready to use.
5. To use the scrub, dampen your skin in the shower then scrub with 1 tablespoon of the scrub mixture.
6. Rinse the scrub away with warm water to leave your skin feeling refreshed.

Cinnamon Honey Lip Scrub

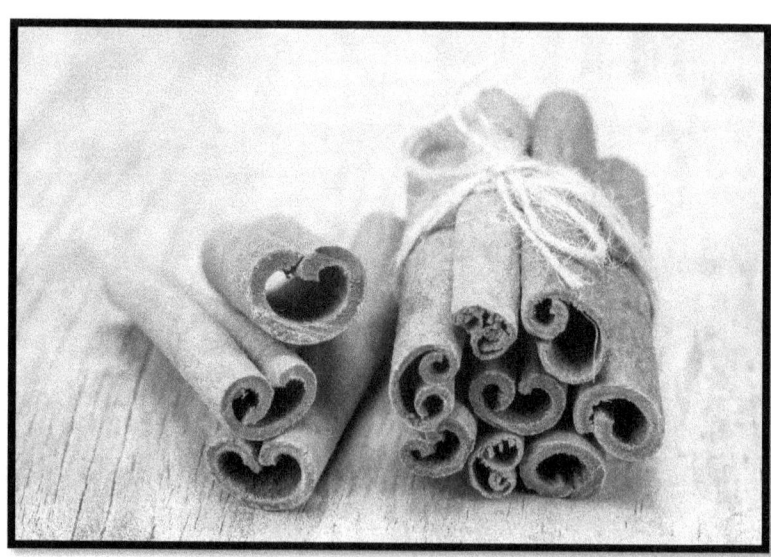

Ingredients:

¼ cup organic brown sugar

1 tablespoon organic coconut oil

1 tablespoon organic raw honey

1 teaspoon organic ground cinnamon

Pinch organic ground cloves

Instructions:

1. Combine the sugar and oil in a small mixing bowl.
2. Stir the ingredients until well combined.
3. Add the remaining ingredients and stir well then transfer to a small glass jar.
4. Place the lid tightly on the jar and store at room temperature until ready to use.
5. To use the scrub, rub a pea-sized amount into your lips in a circular motion for 1 or 2 minutes.
6. Rinse the scrub off with a damp washcloth.

Energizing Coffee Scrub

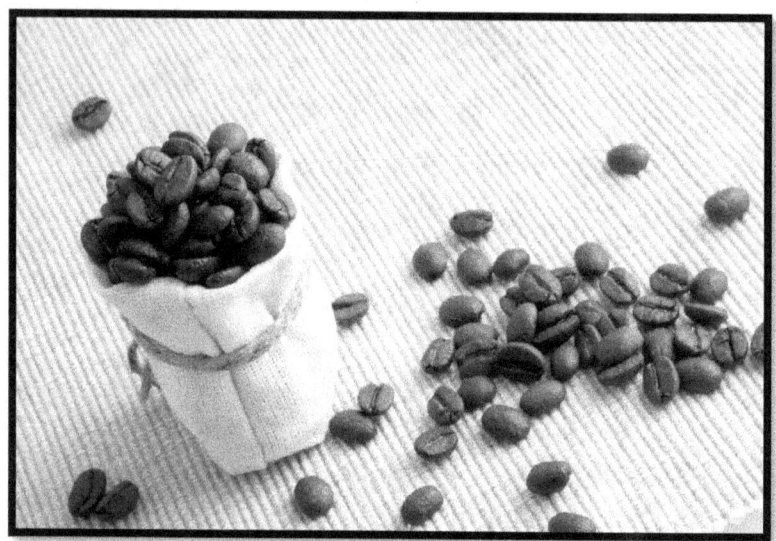

Ingredients:

1 cup organic coconut oil

½ cup organic raw sugar

¼ cup fresh ground coffee

2 ½ tablespoons organic olive oil

Instructions:

1. Combine the sugar and coconut oil in a medium mixing bowl.
2. Stir the ingredients until well combined.

3. Add the remaining ingredients and stir well then transfer to a glass jar.
4. Place the lid tightly on the jar and store at room temperature until ready to use.
5. To use the scrub, dampen your skin in the shower then scrub with 1 tablespoon of the scrub mixture.
6. Rinse the scrub away with warm water to leave your skin feeling refreshed.

Pumpkin Honey Scrub

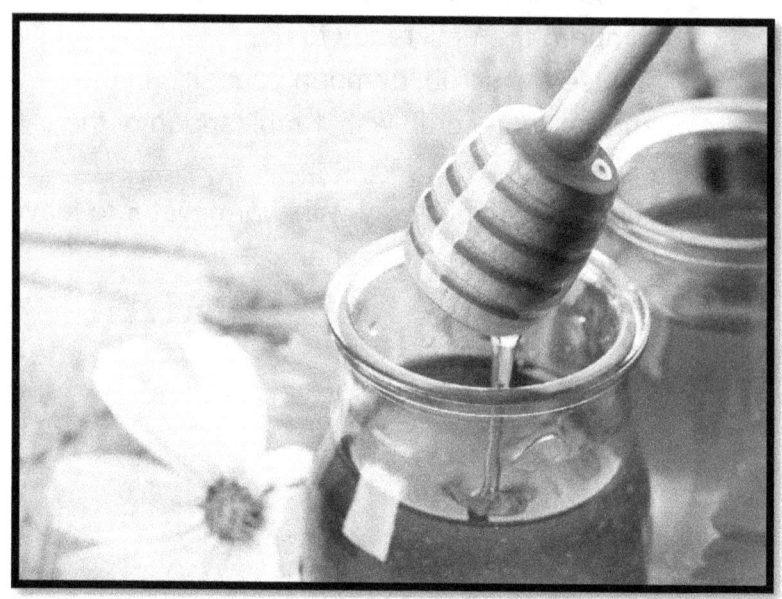

Ingredients:

1 (14 ounce) can organic pumpkin puree

1 cup baking soda

¼ cup organic raw honey

Pinch organic ground cinnamon

Instructions:

1. Combine the pumpkin and baking soda in a medium mixing bowl.
2. Stir the ingredients until well combined.

3. Add the raw honey and cinnamon then stir well then transfer to a glass jar.
4. Place the lid tightly on the jar and store at room temperature until ready to use.
5. To use the scrub, dampen your skin in the shower then scrub with 1 tablespoon of the scrub mixture.
6. Rinse the scrub away with warm water to leave your skin feeling refreshed.

Lemon Coconut Lip Scrub

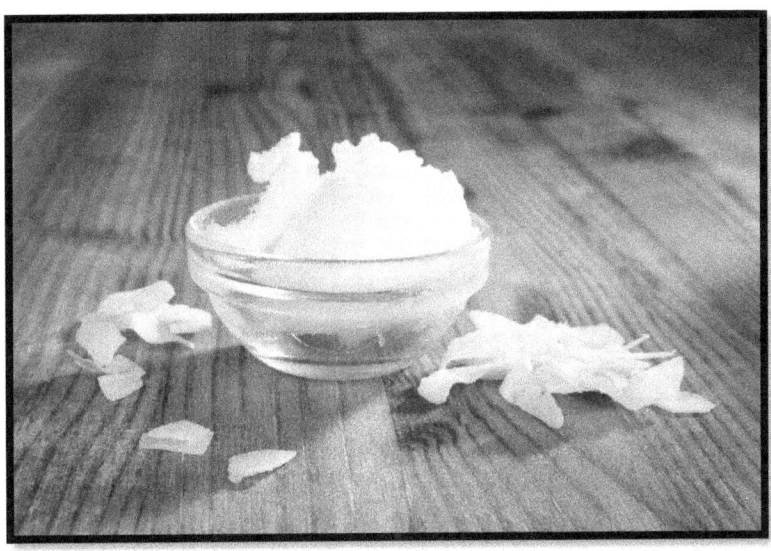

Ingredients:

2 tablespoons organic raw sugar

1 teaspoon organic coconut oil

1 teaspoon organic raw honey

1 teaspoon organic fresh lemon juice

Instructions:

1. Combine the sugar and oil in a small mixing bowl.
2. Stir the ingredients until well combined.
3. Add the remaining ingredients and stir well then transfer to a small glass jar.
4. Place the lid tightly on the jar and store at room temperature until ready to use.
5. To use the scrub, rub a pea-sized amount into your lips in a circular motion for 1 or 2 minutes.
6. Rinse the scrub off with a damp washcloth.

Avocado Grapefruit Scrub

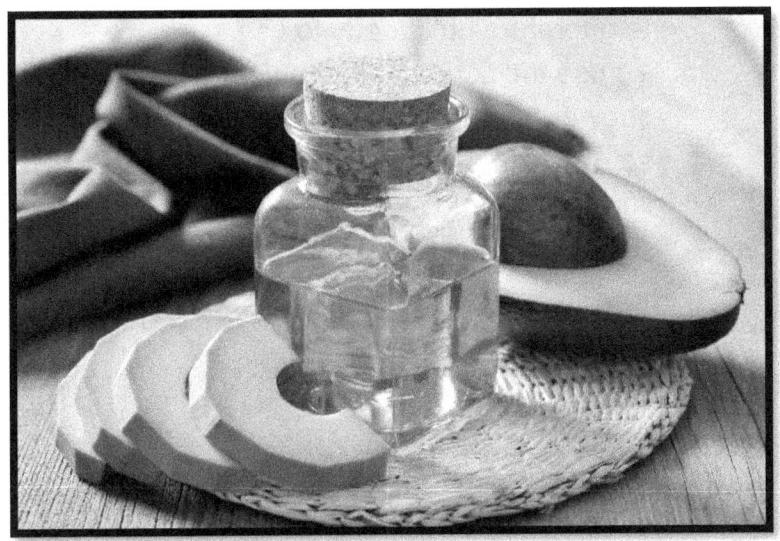

Ingredients:

1 cup organic raw sugar

Juice from ½ raw grapefruit

3 tablespoons organic avocado oil

2 drops organic avocado essential oil

Instructions:

1. Combine the sugar and grapefruit juice in a medium mixing bowl.
2. Stir the ingredients until well combined.

3. Add the remaining ingredients and stir well then transfer to a glass jar.
4. Place the lid tightly on the jar and store at room temperature until ready to use.
5. To use the scrub, dampen your skin in the shower then scrub with 1 tablespoon of the scrub mixture.
6. Rinse the scrub away with warm water to leave your skin feeling refreshed.

Refreshing Lemon Scrub

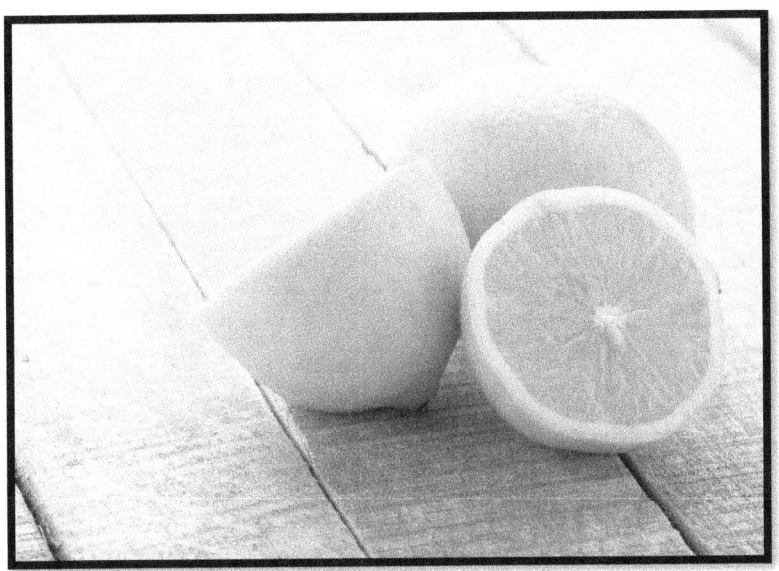

Ingredients:

1 ½ cups organic raw sugar

1/3 cup organic olive oil

1 organic lemon, zested and juiced

1 tablespoon organic vanilla extract

Instructions:

1. Combine the sugar and oil in a medium mixing bowl.
2. Stir the ingredients until well combined.

3. Add the remaining ingredients and stir well then transfer to a glass jar.
4. Place the lid tightly on the jar and store at room temperature until ready to use.
5. To use the scrub, dampen your skin in the shower then scrub with 1 tablespoon of the scrub mixture.
6. Rinse the scrub away with warm water to leave your skin feeling refreshed.

Mint Chocolate Java Lip Scrub

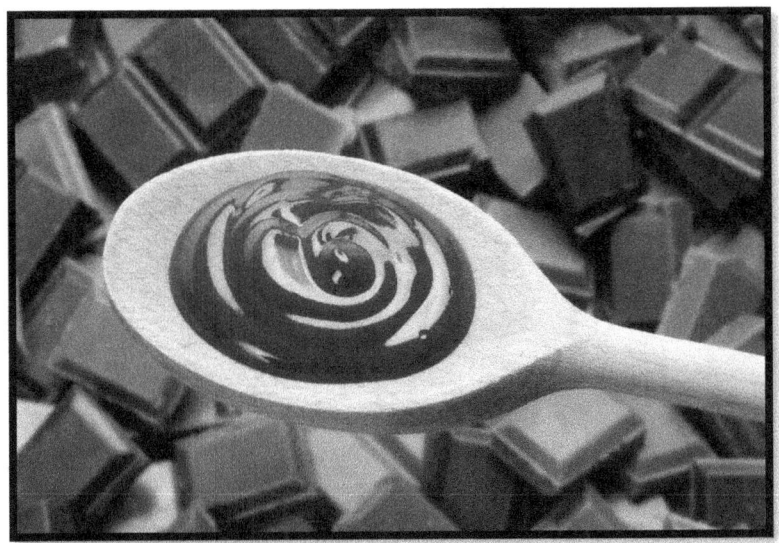

Ingredients:

2 tablespoons organic raw sugar

1 tablespoons organic olive oil

½ teaspoon organic unsweetened cocoa powder

½ teaspoon fresh ground organic coffee beans

2 to 3 drops organic peppermint oil extract

Instructions:

1. Combine the sugar and oil in a small mixing bowl.

2. Stir the ingredients until well combined.
3. Add the remaining ingredients and stir well then transfer to a small glass jar.
4. Place the lid tightly on the jar and store at room temperature until ready to use.
5. To use the scrub, rub a pea-sized amount into your lips in a circular motion for 1 or 2 minutes.
6. Rinse the scrub off with a damp washcloth.

Chocolate Cake Scrub

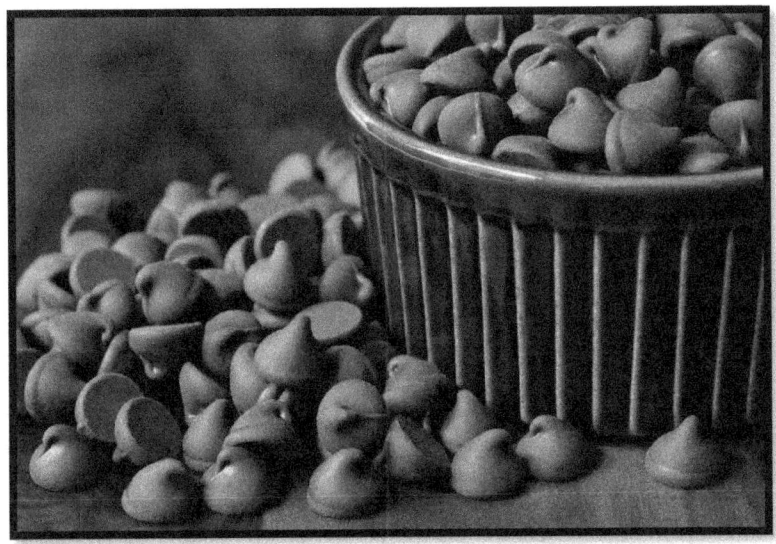

Ingredients:

1 cup organic coconut oil

½ cup organic brown sugar

4 to 5 tablespoons organic unsweetened cocoa powder

½ teaspoon organic vanilla extract

Instructions:

1. Combine the sugar and oil in a medium mixing bowl.
2. Stir the ingredients until well combined.

3. Add the remaining ingredients and stir well then transfer to a glass jar.
4. Place the lid tightly on the jar and store at room temperature until ready to use.
5. To use the scrub, dampen your skin in the shower then scrub with 1 tablespoon of the scrub mixture.
6. Rinse the scrub away with warm water to leave your skin feeling refreshed.

Green Tea and Citrus Scrub

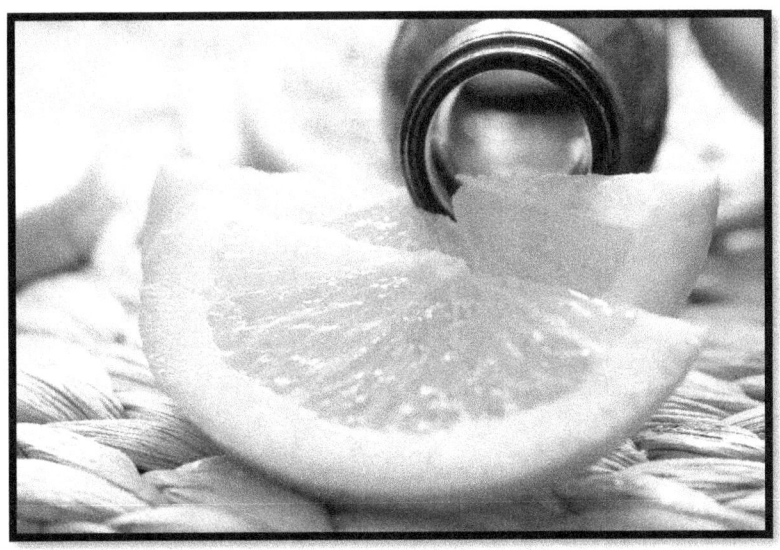

Ingredients:

1 ½ cups Himalayan pink salt (coarse)

1 ½ tablespoons baking soda

2 tablespoons organic grapeseed oil

½ tablespoon loose leaf green tea

3 to 4 drops organic orange essential oil

3 to 4 drops organic lemon essential oil

Zest from 1 organic lime

Instructions:

1. Combine the sea salt and oil in a medium mixing bowl.
2. Stir the ingredients until well combined.
3. Add the remaining ingredients and stir well then transfer to a glass jar.
4. Place the lid tightly on the jar and store at room temperature until ready to use.
5. To use the scrub, dampen your skin in the shower then scrub with 1 tablespoon of the scrub mixture.
6. Rinse the scrub away with warm water to leave your skin feeling refreshed.

Spiced Chai Scrub

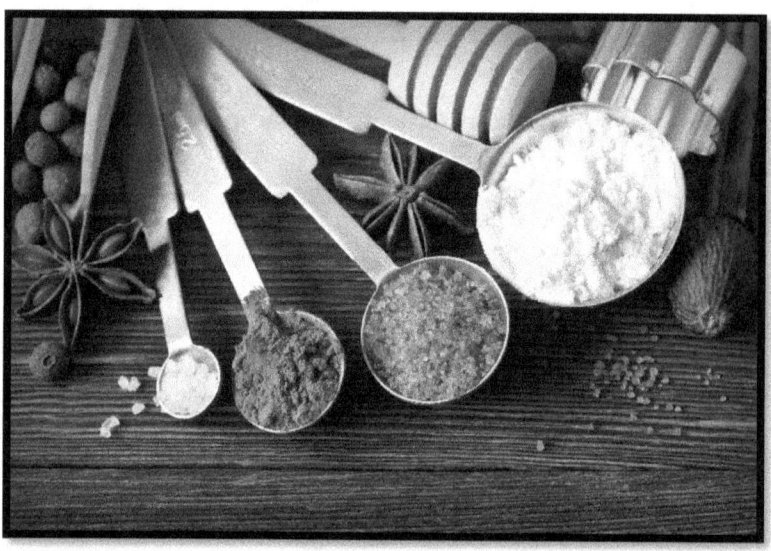

Ingredients:

1 cup organic raw sugar

½ cup organic coconut oil

¼ cup organic black tea

1 tablespoon organic ground ginger

1 tablespoon organic ground cinnamon

1 ½ teaspoons organic vanilla extract

½ teaspoon organic ground nutmeg

½ teaspoon organic ground cloves

¼ teaspoon organic ground cardamom

Pinch organic ground black pepper

Instructions:

1. Combine the sugar and oil in a medium mixing bowl.
2. Stir the ingredients until well combined.
3. Add the remaining ingredients and stir well then transfer to a glass jar.
4. Place the lid tightly on the jar and store at room temperature until ready to use.
5. To use the scrub, dampen your skin in the shower then scrub with 1 tablespoon of the scrub mixture.
6. Rinse the scrub away with warm water to leave your skin feeling refreshed.

Peppermint Lip Scrub

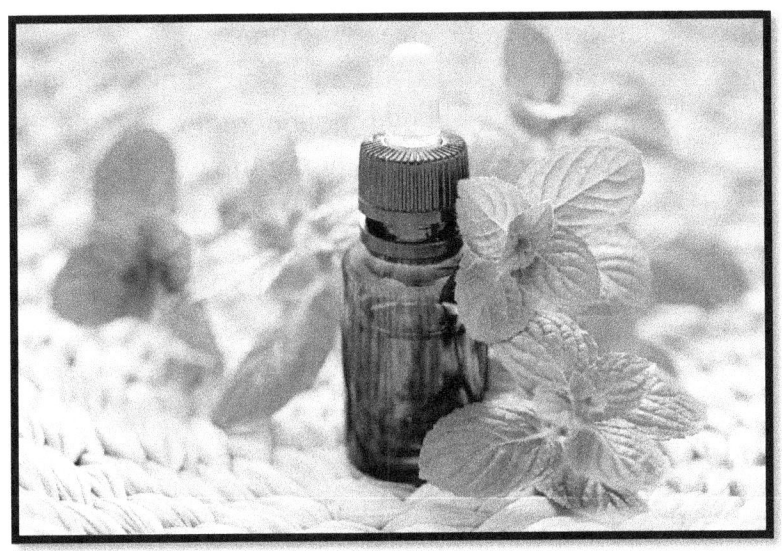

Ingredients:

1 tablespoon organic raw sugar

1 tablespoon organic coconut oil

1 teaspoon organic raw honey

4 to 5 drops organic peppermint essential oil

Instructions:

1. Combine the sugar and oil in a small mixing bowl.
2. Stir the ingredients until well combined.

3. Add the remaining ingredients and stir well then transfer to a small glass jar.
4. Place the lid tightly on the jar and store at room temperature until ready to use.
5. To use the scrub, rub a pea-sized amount into your lips in a circular motion for 1 or 2 minutes.
6. Rinse the scrub off with a damp washcloth.

Coffee Coconut Sugar Scrub

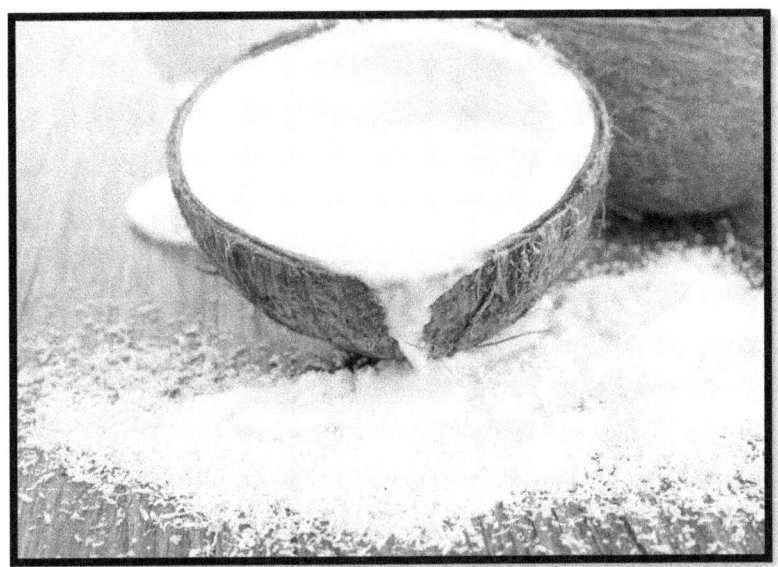

Ingredients:

1 cup organic coconut oil

½ cup organic raw sugar

½ cup organic fresh ground coffee beans

Instructions:

1. Combine the sugar and oil in a medium mixing bowl.
2. Stir the ingredients until well combined.
3. Add the remaining ingredients and stir well then transfer to a glass jar.

4. Place the lid tightly on the jar and store at room temperature until ready to use.
5. To use the scrub, dampen your skin in the shower then scrub with 1 tablespoon of the scrub mixture.
6. Rinse the scrub away with warm water to leave your skin feeling refreshed.

Mint and Pepper Scrub

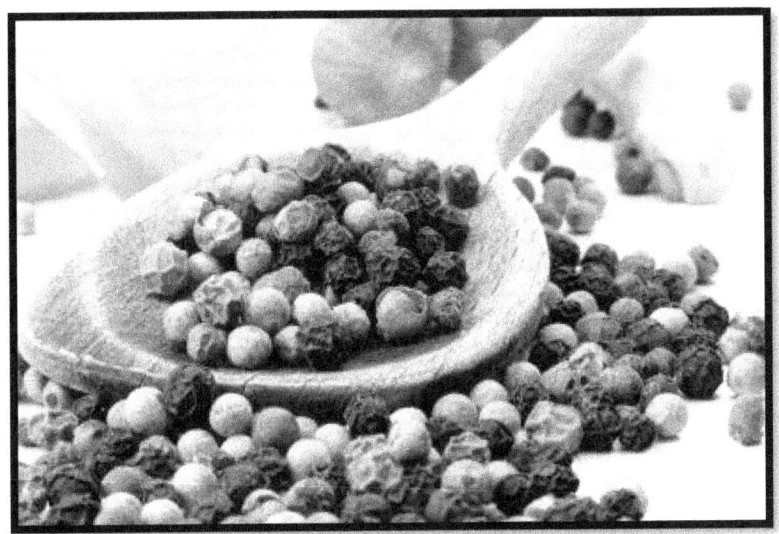

Ingredients:

1 cup Himalayan pink salt (coarse)

½ cup organic olive oil

1 teaspoon organic fresh ground pepper

5 to 6 drops organic mint essential oil

Instructions:

1. Combine the salt and oil in a medium mixing bowl.
2. Stir the ingredients until well combined.

3. Add the remaining ingredients and stir well then transfer to a glass jar.
4. Place the lid tightly on the jar and store at room temperature until ready to use.
5. To use the scrub, dampen your skin in the shower then scrub with 1 tablespoon of the scrub mixture.
6. Rinse the scrub away with warm water to leave your skin feeling refreshed.

Moisturizing Banana Scrub

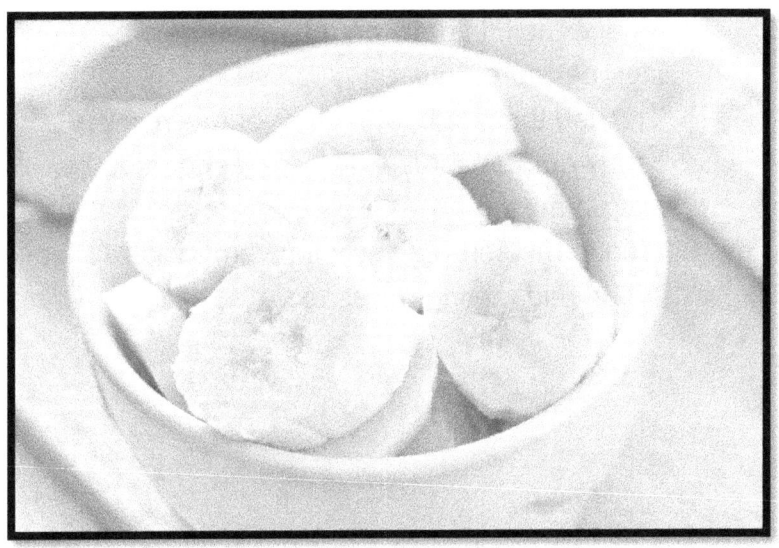

Ingredients:

1 cup organic raw sugar

½ cup organic coconut oil

½ cup organic Shea butter

1 ripe banana, peeled and chopped

Instructions:

1. Combine the sugar and oil in a medium mixing bowl.
2. Stir the ingredients until well combined.

3. Add the remaining ingredients and stir well then transfer to a glass jar – you may also blend them in a food processor.
4. Place the lid tightly on the jar and store at room temperature until ready to use.
5. To use the scrub, dampen your skin in the shower then scrub with 1 tablespoon of the scrub mixture.
6. Rinse the scrub away with warm water to leave your skin feeling refreshed.

Tropical Mango Scrub

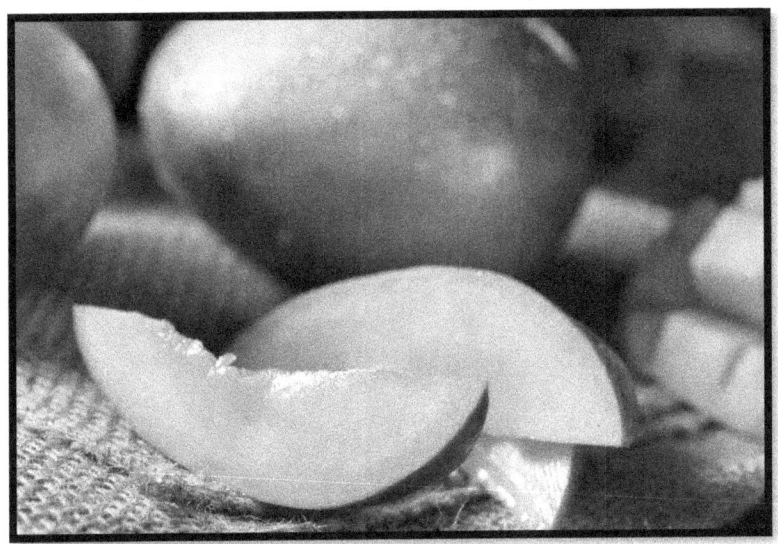

Ingredients:

½ cup organic raw sugar

2 to 3 tablespoons organic coconut oil

¼ cup fresh organic mango, peeled and chopped

4 drops organic orange essential oil

Instructions:

1. Combine the sugar and oil in a medium mixing bowl.
2. Stir the ingredients until well combined.
3. Add the mango and mash it with the spoon.

4. Stir in the essential oil then transfer the ingredients to a glass jar.
5. Place the lid tightly on the jar and store at room temperature until ready to use.
6. To use the scrub, dampen your skin in the shower then scrub with 1 tablespoon of the scrub mixture.
7. Rinse the scrub away with warm water to leave your skin feeling refreshed.

Skin-Soothing Oatmeal Scrub

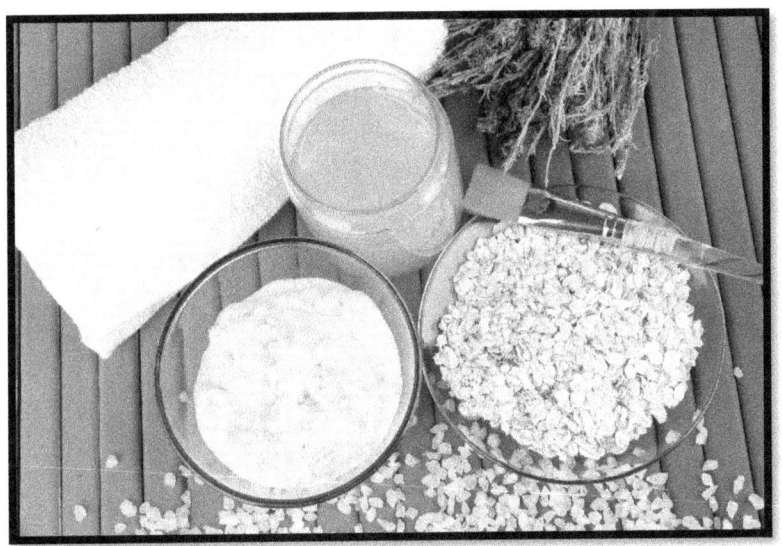

Ingredients:

1 cup organic coconut oil

½ cup organic brown sugar

½ cup organic oatmeal (ground in a food processor)

2 tablespoons organic olive oil

1 teaspoon organic vanilla extract

Instructions:

1. Combine the sugar, oatmeal and oil in a medium mixing bowl.

2. Stir the ingredients until well combined.
3. Add the remaining ingredients and stir well then transfer to a glass jar.
4. Place the lid tightly on the jar and store at room temperature until ready to use.
5. To use the scrub, dampen your skin in the shower then scrub with 1 tablespoon of the scrub mixture.
6. Rinse the scrub away with warm water to leave your skin feeling refreshed.

Mint and Grapefruit Scrub

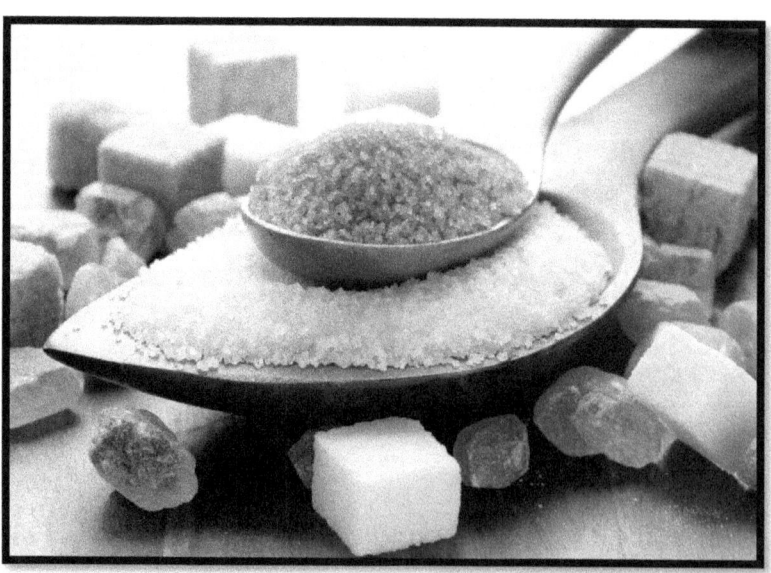

Ingredients:

½ cup organic raw sugar

½ cup organic coconut oil

1 organic grapefruit, zested

1 tablespoon organic grapefruit juice, fresh

8 to 10 drops organic grapefruit essential oil

20 drops organic grapefruit oil

Instructions:

1. Combine the sugar and oil in a medium mixing bowl.
2. Stir the ingredients until well combined.
3. Add the remaining ingredients and stir well then transfer to a glass jar.
4. Place the lid tightly on the jar and store at room temperature until ready to use.
5. To use the scrub, dampen your skin in the shower then scrub with 1 tablespoon of the scrub mixture.
6. Rinse the scrub away with warm water to leave your skin feeling refreshed.

Exfoliating Berry Lip Scrub

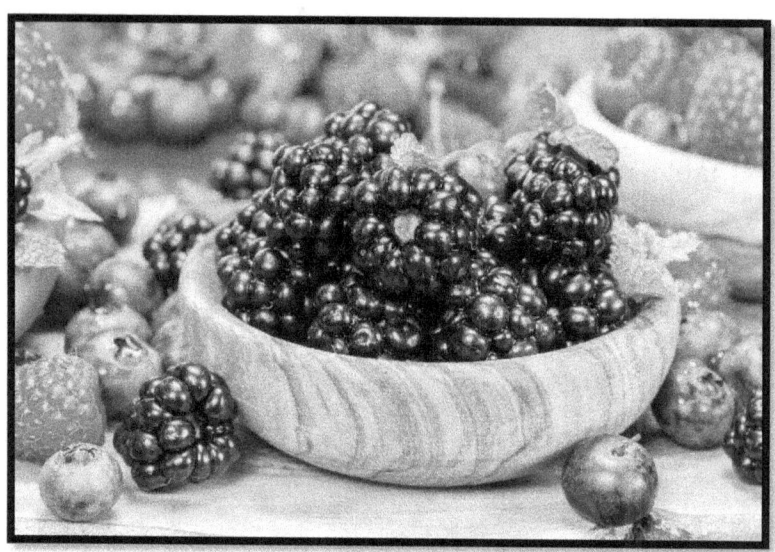

Ingredients:

2 tablespoons organic olive oil

1 ½ teaspoons organic raw sugar

1 teaspoon organic raw honey

1 teaspoon organic fresh lemon juice

2 organic blackberries

Instructions:

1. Combine the honey and oil in a small mixing bowl.

2. Add the berries, crushing them with the spoon and stir the ingredients until well combined.
3. Add the remaining ingredients and stir well then transfer to a small glass jar.
4. Place the lid tightly on the jar and store at room temperature until ready to use.
5. To use the scrub, rub a pea-sized amount into your lips in a circular motion for 1 or 2 minutes.
6. Rinse the scrub off with a damp washcloth.

Brown Sugar Banana Scrub

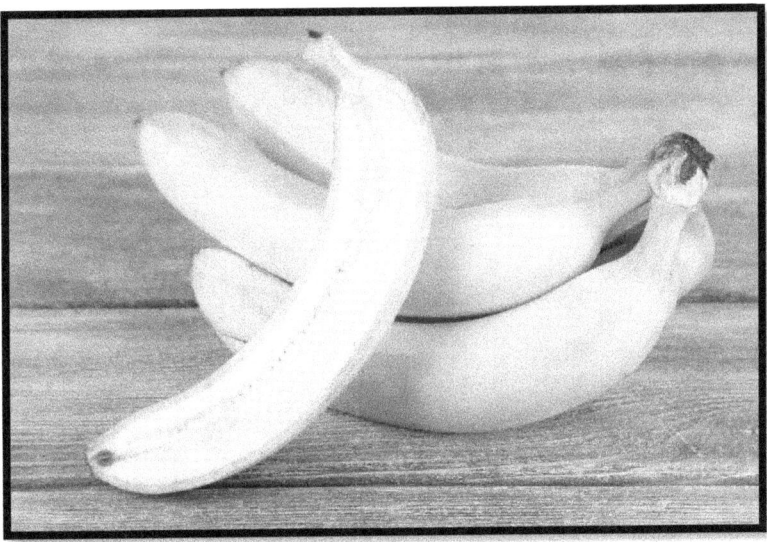

Ingredients:

3 small overripe organic bananas, peeled and chopped

1 cup organic raw brown sugar

Instructions:

1. Combine the bananas and sugar in a medium mixing bowl.
2. Stir the ingredients until well combined then transfer to a glass jar.
3. Place the lid tightly on the jar and store at room temperature until ready to use.
4. To use the scrub, dampen your skin in the shower then scrub with 1 tablespoon of the scrub mixture.
5. Rinse the scrub away with warm water to leave your skin feeling refreshed.

Lavender Sea Salt Scrub

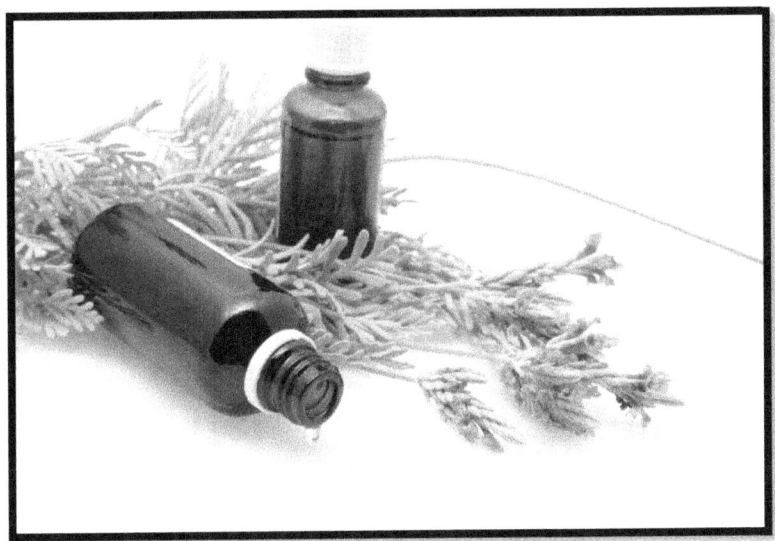

Ingredients:

½ cup Himalayan pink salt (coarse)

1/3 cup organic sweet almond oil

1 tablespoon organic dried lavender

2 to 16 drops organic lavender essential oil

Instructions:

1. Combine the salt and oil in a medium mixing bowl.
2. Stir the ingredients until well combined.

3. Add the remaining ingredients and stir well then transfer to a glass jar.
4. Place the lid tightly on the jar and store at room temperature until ready to use.
5. To use the scrub, dampen your skin in the shower then scrub with 1 tablespoon of the scrub mixture.
6. Rinse the scrub away with warm water to leave your skin feeling refreshed.

Coconut Vanilla Sugar Scrub

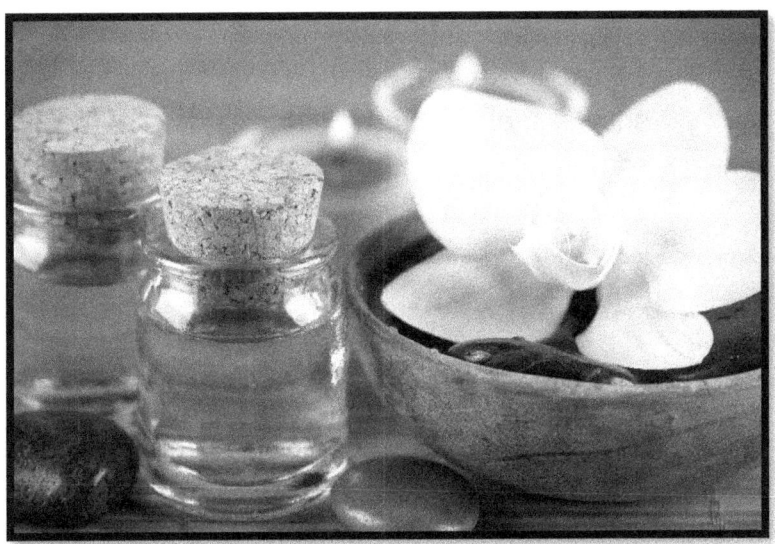

Ingredients:

½ cup organic raw sugar

½ cup organic coconut oil

1 teaspoon organic vanilla extract

3 to 4 drops organic vanilla essential oil

Instructions:

1. Combine the sugar and oil in a medium mixing bowl.
2. Stir the ingredients until well combined.

3. Add the remaining ingredients and stir well then transfer to a glass jar.
4. Place the lid tightly on the jar and store at room temperature until ready to use.
5. To use the scrub, dampen your skin in the shower then scrub with 1 tablespoon of the scrub mixture.
6. Rinse the scrub away with warm water to leave your skin feeling refreshed.

Honey Lime Lip Scrub

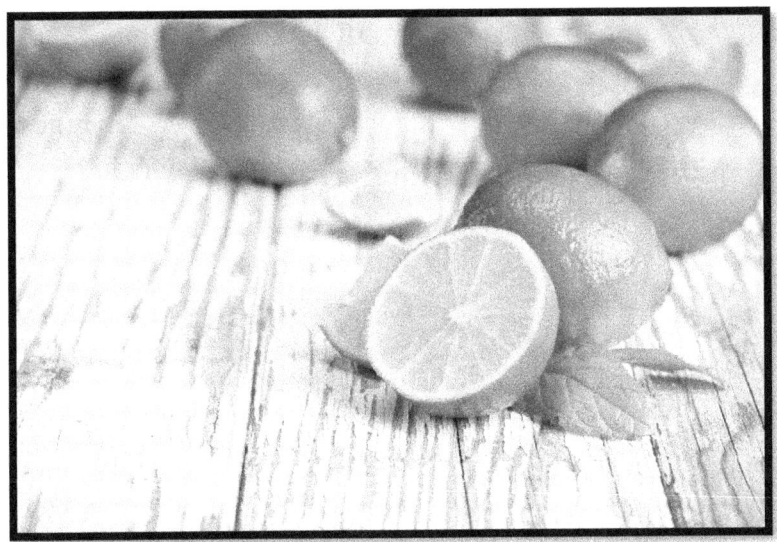

Ingredients:

2 tablespoons organic fresh lime juice

1 tablespoon organic raw sugar

1 tablespoon organic raw honey

2 to 3 drops lime essential oil

Instructions:

1. Combine the sugar and lime juice in a small mixing bowl.
2. Stir the ingredients until well combined.

3. Add the remaining ingredients and stir well then transfer to a small glass jar.
4. Place the lid tightly on the jar and store at room temperature until ready to use.
5. To use the scrub, rub a pea-sized amount into your lips in a circular motion for 1 or 2 minutes.
6. Rinse the scrub off with a damp washcloth.

Rosemary Lemon Salt Scrub

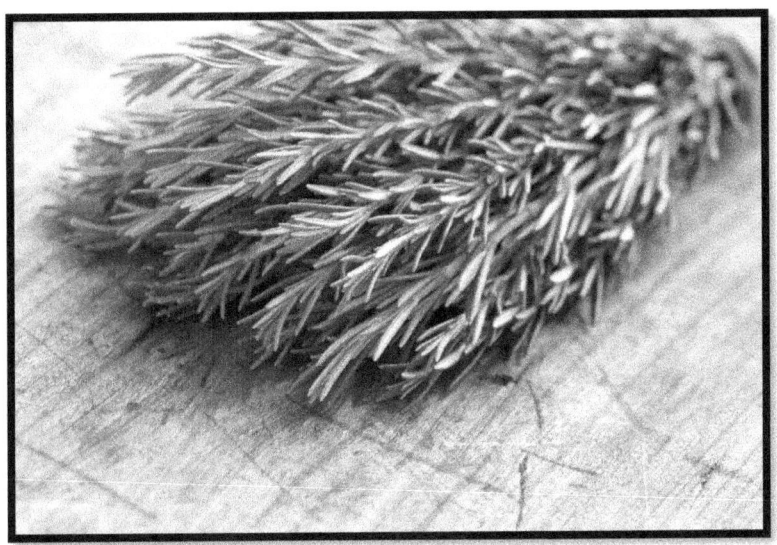

Ingredients:

1 cup Celtic sea salt (coarse)

½ cup organic olive oil

1 organic lemon, zested

2 teaspoons fresh organic rosemary, chopped

3 drops organic rosemary essential oil

Instructions:

1. Combine the salt and oil in a medium mixing bowl.

2. Stir the ingredients until well combined.
3. Add the remaining ingredients and stir well then transfer to a glass jar.
4. Place the lid tightly on the jar and store at room temperature until ready to use.
5. To use the scrub, dampen your skin in the shower then scrub with 1 tablespoon of the scrub mixture.
6. Rinse the scrub away with warm water to leave your skin feeling refreshed.

Ripe Tomato Sugar Scrub

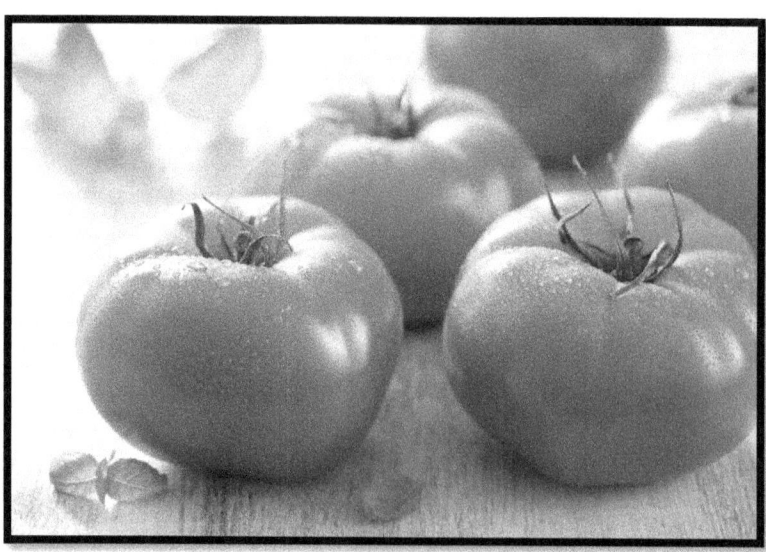

Ingredients:

1 cup organic raw sugar

1/3 cup organic coconut oil

1 small organic Roma tomato, chopped very fine

6 drops organic orange essential oil

6 drops organic lemon essential oil

Instructions:

1. Combine the sugar and oil in a medium mixing bowl.
2. Stir the ingredients until well combined.
3. Add the tomato and mash it with the spoon.
4. Stir in the essential oils then transfer to a glass jar.
5. Place the lid tightly on the jar and store at room temperature until ready to use.
6. To use the scrub, dampen your skin in the shower then scrub with 1 tablespoon of the scrub mixture.
7. Rinse the scrub away with warm water to leave your skin feeling refreshed.

Minty Sugar Lip Scrub

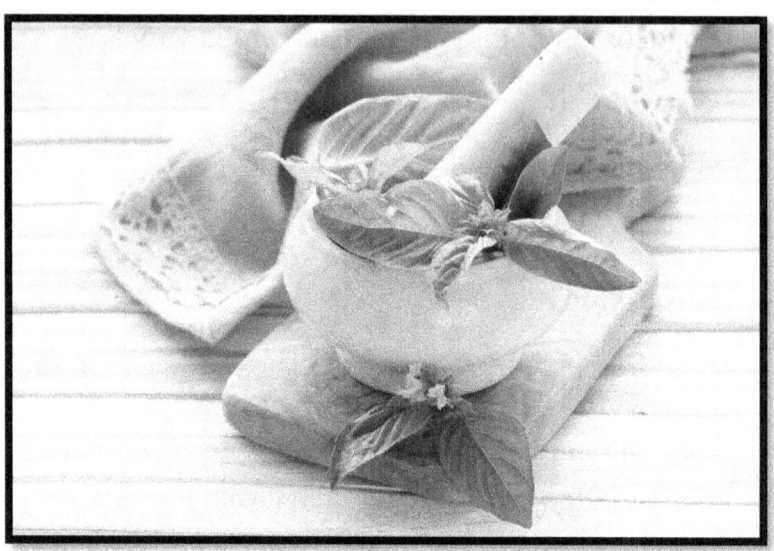

Ingredients:

1 tablespoon organic raw sugar

1 tablespoon organic olive oil

1 teaspoon organic raw agave

4 to 5 drops organic mint essential oil

Instructions:

1. Combine the sugar and oil in a small mixing bowl.
2. Stir the ingredients until well combined.

3. Add the remaining ingredients and stir well then transfer to a small glass jar.
4. Place the lid tightly on the jar and store at room temperature until ready to use.
5. To use the scrub, rub a pea-sized amount into your lips in a circular motion for 1 or 2 minutes.
6. Rinse the scrub off with a damp washcloth.

Orange Sea Salt Scrub

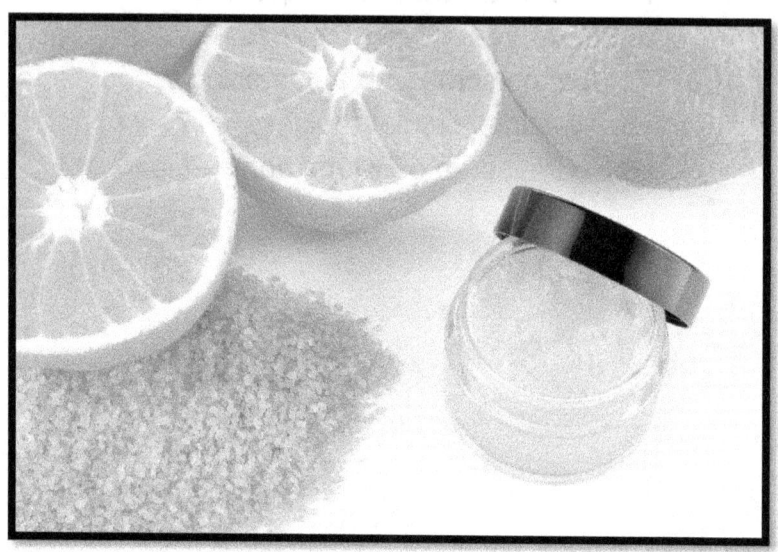

Ingredients:

½ cup Celtic sea salt (coarse)

½ cup organic olive oil

1 teaspoon organic orange zest

4 to 6 drops organic orange essential oil

Instructions:

1. Combine the salt and oil in a medium mixing bowl.
2. Stir the ingredients until well combined.

3. Add the remaining ingredients and stir well then transfer to a glass jar.
4. Place the lid tightly on the jar and store at room temperature until ready to use.
5. To use the scrub, dampen your skin in the shower then scrub with 1 tablespoon of the scrub mixture.
6. Rinse the scrub away with warm water to leave your skin feeling refreshed.

Vanilla Brown Sugar Scrub

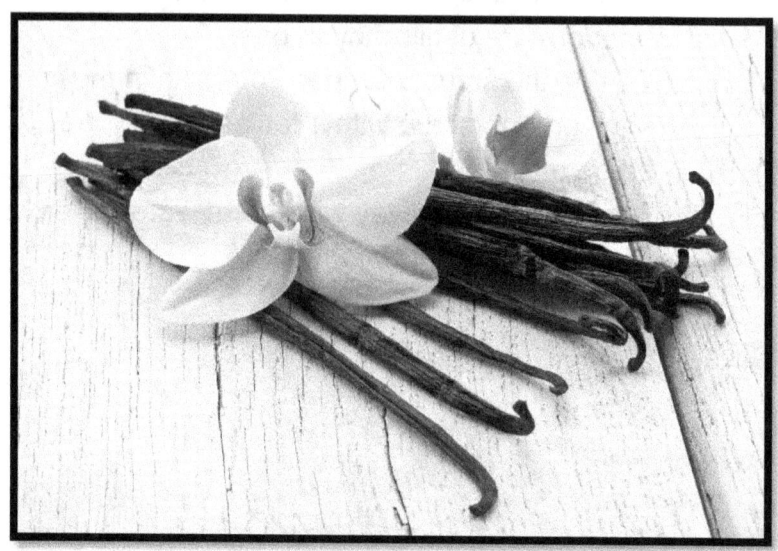

Ingredients:

1 ½ cups organic raw brown sugar

½ cup organic olive oil

2 teaspoons organic vanilla extract

8 to 12 drops organic vanilla essential oil

Instructions:

1. Combine the sugar and oil in a medium mixing bowl.
2. Stir the ingredients until well combined.

3. Add the remaining ingredients and stir well then transfer to a glass jar.
4. Place the lid tightly on the jar and store at room temperature until ready to use.
5. To use the scrub, dampen your skin in the shower then scrub with 1 tablespoon of the scrub mixture.
6. Rinse the scrub away with warm water to leave your skin feeling refreshed.

Lemon Raspberry Sugar Scrub

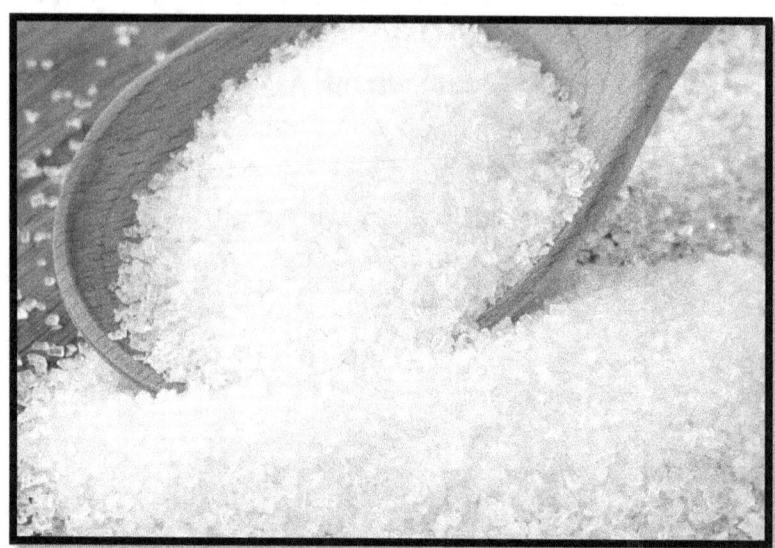

Ingredients:

1 cup organic raw sugar

¼ cup organic coconut oil, melted

12 drops organic lemon essential oil

15 drops organic raspberry essential oil

3 to 4 drops red food coloring (optional)

Instructions:

1. Combine the sugar and oil in a medium mixing bowl.

2. Stir the ingredients until well combined.
3. Add the remaining ingredients and stir well then transfer to a glass jar.
4. Place the lid tightly on the jar and store at room temperature until ready to use.
5. To use the scrub, dampen your skin in the shower then scrub with 1 tablespoon of the scrub mixture.
6. Rinse the scrub away with warm water to leave your skin feeling refreshed.

Conclusion

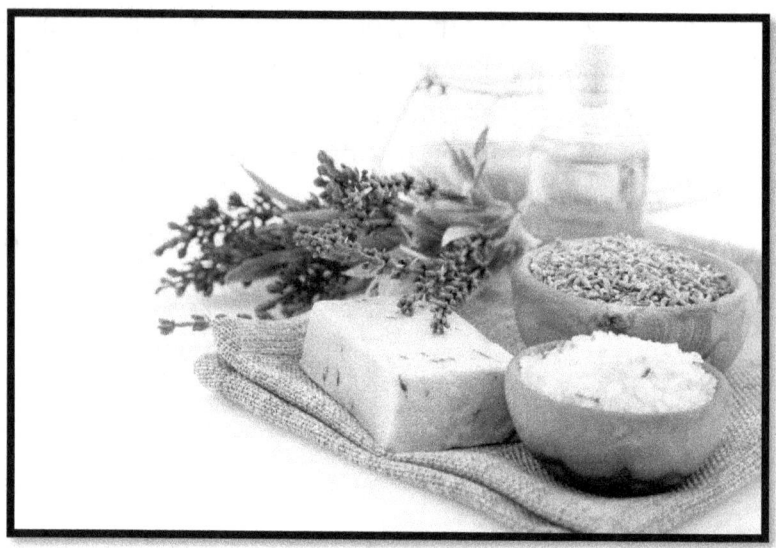

Never again will you have to spend a small fortune at the spa for special organic body scrubs. With just a few simple ingredients, you can make your own organic body scrubs at home! Ingredients like coconut oil, raw sugar, and essential oils are all that you need to get started and there are an endless number of combinations you can try. If you are ready to start making your own organic body scrubs at home, pick a recipe from this book and give it a try!

I Need Your Help!

Please take a minute out of your busy schedule to leave a review.

Your review will let readers know what to expect and what you liked about this book. I am looking forward to reading your review.

Thank you so much for your feedback!

www.ingramcontent.com/pod-product-compliance
Lightning Source LLC
Chambersburg PA
CBHW070819290526
45795CB00002B/763